SIMPLE MORNING WORKOUTS FOR MEN

9 minutes a day simple fitness exercise for Weight loss, improved cardiovascular health, balance and flexibility for improved Body health

David B. Manning

TABLE OF CONTENT

INTRODUCTION

Tobey, a lively man full of energy and excitement, encountered unanticipated obstacles that jeopardized his health. Despite his enthusiasm for life, his sedentary profession and lifestyle were taking a toll on his physique.

Hours spent sitting at a desk have resulted in a lack of flexibility, stiffness in his knees, and persistent back discomfort. Tobey acknowledged the need for change after becoming aware of the possible problems that his lifestyle may present.

Concerned about his cardiovascular health, extra body weight, and increased exhaustion, Tobey set out on a journey to restore his well-being. He understood that adopting preemptive action was critical to avoiding the impending health concerns. In his search for remedies, Tobey came upon Simple Morning Workouts for Men.

The book was a revelation, with precise exercises that addressed Tobey's individual concerns. With resolve and a renewed sense of purpose, Tobey started incorporating the workouts into his everyday regimen. What began as a timid endeavor quickly evolved into a steadfast dedication to self-improvement.

As the days progressed into weeks, Tobey observed substantial changes in both his body and psyche. The rigid joints began to soften, allowing him to move with greater ease and elegance.

The constant back ache reduced with time, giving way to a sense of strength and perseverance. With each passing day, Tobey felt more invigorated and vibrant than before.

However, the shift extended beyond physical health. Tobey's mental clarity and happiness improved as he adopted a more active lifestyle. The mere act of moving his body became a source of joy and fulfillment, feeding his love of life in ways he never expected.

Tobey's devotion and tenacity not only restored his health, but also gave him a renewed feeling of vigor and purpose. Armed with the information and resources included within the pages of Simple Morning Workouts for Men.

Chapter 1: Benefits of Morning Exercise

Morning exercise has several benefits to males, including establishing a favorable tone for the day ahead. Here's a detailed look at why including easy morning workouts into your regimen might be beneficial.

Morning exercise boosts your metabolism, allowing you to burn more calories throughout the day. This can help with weight control and fat loss objectives.

Improves Mood: Morning exercises cause the body to produce endorphins, which are natural mood boosters. Starting your day with exercise may elevate your spirits, reduce stress, and boost your sense of pleasure and well-being.

Increases Energy Levels: Instead of grabbing for a cup of coffee, try a morning workout to revitalize your body. Exercise improves blood circulation and oxygen flow, delivering a natural energy boost to get through the day's chores.

Exercise boosts brain activity, which improves mental clarity and concentration. Working exercise in the morning sets a favorable tone for productivity, helping you to remain alert and focused throughout the day.

Promotes greater Sleep: Regular morning exercise can help regulate your sleep-wake cycle, resulting in greater quality sleep at night. This guarantees you wake up feeling rejuvenated and ready to face the day.

Strengthens Immune System: A consistent morning exercise regimen can boost your immune system, making you less vulnerable to diseases and infections. It helps the body eliminate pollutants, keeping you healthy and robust.

Builds Discipline and Routine: Adding early workouts to your regular routine instills discipline and promotes healthy behaviors. It establishes a precedent for valuing self-care and physical well-being, resulting in long-term health advantages.

Improves Confidence and Self-esteem: Regular exercise might help you feel better about your physique. Starting your day with an exercise sets a good tone, increasing confidence and self-assurance.

Improves Heart Health: Morning exercise strengthens the heart and cardiovascular system, which lowers the risk of heart disease and stroke. It also helps to manage blood pressure and cholesterol levels, therefore improving overall heart health.

Increases lifespan: Research has revealed that regular exercise is associated with enhanced lifespan. Incorporating morning workouts into your schedule is an investment in your long-term health and well-being.

Simple morning workouts for men have several advantages, including physical, mental, and emotional well-being. Making exercise a priority in the morning prepares you for a productive, invigorated, and joyful day ahead.

Overcoming Barriers

Adding early exercises to your schedule may be revolutionary, but it is not without hurdles.

Whether it's the challenge of getting up early or finding time in a hectic schedule, overcoming obstacles is critical for continuous exercise. Here's a thorough guide on overcoming barriers and adopting basic morning workouts for men:

Set Clear Goals: Define your fitness targets and divide them into manageable milestones. Knowing your goals will offer you drive and direction.

Create a routine: Set a regular wake-up time and adhere to it, even on weekends. A planned regimen regulates your body's internal clock, making it simpler to get up early.

Begin Slowly: If you're not used to morning exercises, ease into it. Begin with shorter workouts and gradually increase the intensity and length as your body adapts.

Prepare the Night Before: Lay out your exercise clothing, fill your water bottle, and set up any necessary equipment the night before. This reduces friction in the morning and eliminates excuses.

Find Accountability: Hold yourself accountable by partnering with a buddy or joining a morning workout group. Knowing that someone depends on you may be a great incentive.

Focus on Consistency, Not Perfection: Don't beat yourself up if you skip one or two workouts. The most important thing is to be consistent throughout time. Aim for growth, not perfection.

Fuel Your Body: Eat a small snack or a pre-workout meal to give your body the energy it requires. To properly feed your workout, choose a combination of carbs and protein.

Mix It Up: Make your morning workouts more entertaining by adding a range of exercises and activities. This reduces boredom and helps to target different muscle areas.

Listen to your body. Pay attention to how your body reacts to early exercises and modify accordingly. Rest as required and avoid pushing through discomfort or tiredness.

Celebrate Progress: Recognize your accomplishments, no matter how minor. Recognizing your progress promotes morale and encourages good behaviors.

By breaking down barriers and adopting basic morning workouts for guys, you will not only improve your physical health, but also your well-being and productivity throughout the day.

With effort and perseverance, you may transform morning exercise into a gratifying element of your daily routine.

Setting Goals

Setting objectives is critical for success in any pursuit, including adding basic morning workouts to your regimen. Setting specific and attainable goals can help you stay motivated, measure your progress, and eventually achieve your fitness goals.

First, determine your fitness goals. Be explicit about your goals, whether they are to lose weight, gain muscle, increase stamina, or improve general health. This clarity can help direct your training routine and keep you focused.

Next, create a realistic timeframe. Setting short- and long-term objectives enables you to divide your fitness journey into digestible chunks. For example, set a goal to lose a certain amount of weight in three months or raise your strength by a specific percentage in six months.

Adjust your goals as appropriate to reflect your progress and any changes in circumstances.

Once you've established your goals, build a fitness schedule that is specific to your requirements and tastes. Given the restricted amount of time and energy available, early workouts should be basic yet effective.

Choose activities that target many muscular groups at once, such as bodyweight exercises, circuit training, or high-intensity interval training (HIIT).

Consistency is essential for accomplishing fitness objectives. Make a commitment to stick to your morning fitness program, even if you don't feel like it.

Making exercise a non-negotiable part of your daily plan can help you develop momentum and see improvements over time.

Tracking your success is critical for maintaining motivation and accountability. Keep an exercise log or utilize fitness apps to document your workouts, performance, and progress toward your objectives.

Celebrate your accomplishments along the road, whether it's setting a new personal best or keeping to a steady training schedule.

Maintain flexibility and adjust your goals and training regimen as required. Life is unpredictable, and circumstances may change, so be prepared to modify your approach appropriately.

Remember that setbacks are a normal part of the process; the most important thing is to remain dedicated and keep pushing forward.

Setting objectives is critical for success when implementing basic morning workouts into your regimen.

You may improve your fitness and general well-being by defining clear goals, setting a realistic schedule, designing a specific training plan, keeping consistent, measuring your progress, and remaining adaptable.

Chapter 2: Warm-up and Mobility

Warm-up and mobility exercises are essential components of every training plan, especially for men who begin their day with basic morning workouts.

These warm-up exercises not only serve to prevent injuries, but they also improve performance by boosting blood flow to the muscles and joint flexibility. Here's a detailed guide for adding warm-up and mobility exercises to your morning routine:

Dynamic Stretching: Start with activities like arm circles, leg swings, and torso twists. These movements engage the muscles and lubricate the joints, getting them ready for more strenuous action.

Foam rolling: Use a foam roller to target tight muscles and relieve stress. Focus on the calves, hamstrings, quadriceps, and upper back. Roll carefully and deliberately, stopping on any tender areas to provide mild pressure.

Joint Mobilization: Do movements to mobilize important joints, such as shoulder circles, wrist circles, hip circles, and ankle circles. This improves joint range of motion and reduces the chance of damage during exercise.

Dynamic Warm-up: Perform a series of dynamic warm-up activities to help engage the muscles and raise your heart rate.

Examples include high knees, butt kicks, walking lunges, and inchworms. Aim to progressively raise the intensity to get the body ready for more intense action.

Planks, bird dogs, and abdominal crunches are examples of exercises that can help you engage your core muscles. A strong core offers stability and support throughout workouts, lowering the chance of injury and increasing overall performance.

Balance and Stability: Include balance and stability exercises in your warm-up routine to improve proprioception and coordination. Single-leg balances, heel-to-toe walks, and stability ball exercises can help you improve your balance and functional movement patterns.

Spend a few seconds focusing on deep, conscious breathing. Inhale deeply via the nose to fill the lungs with air, then gently exhale through the mouth. This helps to relax the mind, relieve tension, and mentally prepare for the upcoming workout.

By devoting only a few minutes each morning to warm-up and mobility exercises, men may improve their performance, avoid injuries, and lay the groundwork for a productive day. Include these easy yet powerful strategies in your morning routine to gain the advantages of a strong and healthy body.

Importance of Warm-up

Warm-up activities are essential in every fitness plan, including basic morning workouts for guys. These first motions get the body ready for more intense exercises by gradually raising heart rate, circulation, and flexibility. Here's why warming up is essential for men starting their early workouts:

Warm-up activities, which progressively increase blood flow to muscles and joints, can lower the risk of injury during future physical activity. Warming up relaxes tight muscles, making them less susceptible to strains and rips.

Improved Performance: A thorough warm-up prepares the body for exercise, which boosts performance throughout the exercise. It lets muscles contract more effectively, resulting in increased strength, power and endurance. Men who warm up properly tend to do better in their exercises, whether they are lifting weights, running, or participating in sports activities.

Enhanced Flexibility: Morning workouts frequently follow a period of inactivity while sleeping, leaving muscles tight and stiff. Warm-up activities help to develop flexibility by lengthening muscles and enhancing joint mobility. This not only decreases the danger of damage, but also provides a wider range of motion during activities.

Warming up not only prepares men physically, but also mentally for the trials that lie ahead. It helps shift emphasis from morning grogginess to the next workout, increasing motivation and mental clarity. This mental preparation might result in a more effective and concentrated training session.

Improved Circulation: During sleep, circulation slows, resulting in less blood supply to muscles and organs. A warm-up increases circulation, supplying oxygen and nutrients to muscles while eliminating waste. This improves energy production and metabolism, giving the fuel required for a morning workout.

Simple morning workouts for guys might include a variety of warm-up activities including dynamic stretches, mild cardio, and mobility drills.

These activities should gradually increase in intensity while mimicking the motions of the impending workout. Warm-up activities lasting 5-10 minutes can considerably improve the efficacy and safety of morning workouts.

Warm-up activities are vital for guys beginning their morning workouts. They not only lower the chance of injury, but also boost performance, flexibility, and mental preparedness. Men may get the most out of

their early workout routine by implementing
a thorough warm-up program.

Dynamic Stretches

Dynamic stretches are an important part of any training regimen, especially in the morning, because they help your body prepare for physical activity and lower the chance of injury.

Unlike static stretches, which entail holding a posture for a lengthy amount of time, dynamic stretches feature constant movement that simulates the motions you'll do during your workout.

For guys seeking a quick morning workout regimen, dynamic stretches can be really useful. These stretches promote not just flexibility, but also blood flow, muscle activation, and overall performance.

To begin your morning routine, do a quick warm-up such as running in place or jumping jacks to get your blood flowing. After warming up, incorporate dynamic stretches that target key muscle groups, such as:

Leg Swings: Stand tall and swing one leg forward and backward, gradually expanding your range of motion. This stretch relaxes the hamstrings, quadriceps, and hip flexors.

Arm Circles: Extend your arms to the sides and perform circular motions, progressively increasing in diameter. Arm circles assist to release the shoulders and upper back.

Torso Twists: Stand with your feet hip-width apart, then twist your torso from side to side while engaging your core. This stretch moves the spine and activates the obliques.

Hip Circles: Stand with your feet hip-width apart and move your hips in circular motions, progressively increasing the size of each circle. This stretch increases hip mobility and loosens the hip flexors.

Lunges with Rotation: Step forward into a lunge stance, then rotate your torso toward the front leg.

Do same thing on the other side and return to the starting point This stretch increases hip flexibility and engages core muscles.

Perform each vigorous stretch 10-15 times or for roughly 30 seconds on each side. Maintain good form and control during all motions.

Incorporating dynamic stretches into your morning routine not only gets your body ready for the day, but it also sets a good tone for your overall health and fitness objectives.

listen to your body and alter the intensity of the stretches accordingly. With practice, you'll notice more flexibility, less muscular tension, and better performance in your exercises and daily tasks.

Foam Rolling Techniques

Foam rolling is a simple yet powerful practice for relieving muscular tension, increasing flexibility, and hastening recovery. Incorporating foam rolling into your morning workout regimen will help you feel refreshed and ready to face the day's difficulties. Here's a complete guide on foam rolling methods designed for men's morning workouts:

Start with a Warm-Up: Before foam rolling, you should warm up your muscles with some mild aerobic or dynamic stretches. This prepares your muscles for the rolling motion and boosts blood flow to the targeted locations.

Foam roll major muscular areas first, such as the calves, quadriceps, hamstrings, glutes, and back.

Before rolling back and forth slowly,spend 1-2 minutes on each muscle

Apply the Proper Pressure: Adjust the pressure on the foam roller based on your degree of comfort and the intensity of muscle tightness. You should feel some discomfort, but not too much agony.

Use Long, Fluid Strokes: Roll each muscle group from the origin to the muscle's insertion point. This breaks up adhesions and knots while improving circulation.

Target specific areas: Pay special attention to regions that are extremely tight or uncomfortable, such as the IT band, hip flexors, and shoulders. Spend more time on these regions to relieve tension and increase mobility.

Breathe and Relax: Remember to take deep breaths and relax your muscles when foam rolling. Tension or holding your breath might reduce the effectiveness of the approach.

Incorporate Trigger Points: If you come across a particularly delicate region, known as a trigger point, pause and apply mild pressure for 20-30 seconds until you feel the tension subside.

Finish with Stretching: After foam rolling, perform static stretches to improve flexibility and range of motion in the muscles you targeted.

Hydrate and Refuel: Following your morning workout, drink lots of water to rehydrate your body and restore lost nutrients. Consider having a nutritious breakfast to jumpstart your metabolism and power your day.

Incorporating these foam rolling techniques into your easy morning routines will help you enhance muscle function, lower your chance of injury, and perform better all day long. Make foam rolling a regular part of your workout program to reap the most advantages and improve your fitness journey.

Chapter 3: Strength Training

Strength training is an essential component of any fitness regimen, particularly for men who want to gain muscle growth, boost strength, and improve overall health.

Simple morning workouts may be a great way to include strength training into your daily routine and establish a good tone for the rest of the day. Here's a complete guide to basic morning strength training programs for men.

Warm-up: Begin with a quick warm-up to prepare your muscles and joints for the forthcoming activity. Arm circles, leg swings, and torso twists are excellent stretches for releasing tight muscles and improving blood flow.

Bodyweight Exercises: Incorporate push-ups, squats, lunges, and planks into your morning workout. These movements train numerous muscle groups at the same time, giving you a whole-body workout without the use of any equipment.

Progressive Overload: As you grow more comfortable with bodyweight exercises, gradually raise the intensity by including variations or doing more repetitions. Steady stress promotes muscular growth and strength development over time.

Resistance Bands: To add resistance to your early exercises, utilize resistance bands. Exercises such as banded squats, bicep curls, and lateral raises can efficiently target particular muscle areas while increasing overall strength.

Dumbbell Exercises: If you can access dumbbells, incorporate dumbbell presses, rows, deadlifts, and curls in your morning workout. Dumbbells have adjustable resistance so that you may tune the intensity of your workout to your fitness level.

Circuit Training: To improve efficiency, organize your morning exercises into circuit training sessions. To keep your heart rate high and burn the most calories, alternate between different exercises with little breaks between sets.

Cool down: After your morning workout, spend a few minutes stretching your muscles. This helps to avoid injury, minimize muscular pain, and increase flexibility and mobility.

Consistency is essential for seeing benefits from your early strength training routines. Aim to exercise three to four times per week, gradually increasing the intensity and length of your workouts as you progress.

By incorporating simple morning strength training workouts into your routine, you can gain muscle, increase strength, and improve overall health and fitness. With dedication and consistency, you'll soon reap the benefits of a stronger, more resilient body, laying the groundwork for a productive day.

Bodyweight Exercises

Bodyweight exercises are a simple and efficient approach for men to start their days with a boost of energy and fitness. These exercises use the body's own weight as resistance and need minimum equipment and space, making them ideal for home training. Here's a full list of basic morning bodyweight workouts for men:

1. *Push-Ups:* Start your morning workout with a set of push-ups to work your chest, shoulders, and triceps. Begin with a manageable amount of reps and progressively increase as you gain strength.

2. *Squats:* Squats are great for increasing lower-body strength and stability. Stand with your feet shoulder-width apart, then drop your hips back and down as if sitting in a chair, before returning to standing posture. Aim for good form and controlled motions.

3. *Lunges:* Lunges engage several muscle groups, including the quadriceps, glutes, and hamstrings.

With both knees Bent at a 90-degree angle, Move forward with one leg and lowering your hip.

Then return to standing and repeat with the opposite leg.

4. *Planks:* These exercises help to strengthen your core muscles. Begin in a push-up posture, then drop onto your forearms while keeping your body in a straight line from head to heels. Hold for 30-60 seconds, making sure your abs are engaged and your hips remain level.

5. *Mountain Climbers:* This dynamic workout works the core, shoulders, and legs while increasing cardiovascular fitness. Begin in a plank posture, then alternately raise each knee to your chest in a running motion.

6. *Burpees:* A full-body workout that combines strength and cardio. Begin in a standing posture, then stoop down, lay your hands on the ground, leap your feet back into a plank, do a push-up, jump your feet back to your hands, and burst upward into a jump.

7. *Jumping Jacks:* Finish your morning workout with some jumping jacks to raise your heart rate and enhance circulation. Jump your feet out wide, lifting your arms high, and then return to the starting position.

Add these bodyweight exercises to your morning routine for a quick and effective approach to improve your strength, stamina, and general health. Begin with a moderate amount of reps, gradually increasing intensity as you advance.

To avoid injury, maintain appropriate form and listen to your body. With regularity and devotion, you'll quickly see the results of a healthier, stronger physique.

Dumbbell/Kettlebell Workouts

Dumbbell and kettlebell workouts are a diverse and efficient approach for men to begin their mornings with a brief yet significant fitness program.

These little pieces of equipment may be readily integrated into easy morning exercises, delivering a full-body workout that targets numerous muscle groups while also increasing cardiovascular health, general strength, and endurance.

One of the primary advantages of combining dumbbell and kettlebell workouts into morning routines is their effectiveness. Men may work many muscle groups at the same time with only a few sets of exercises, maximizing their limited time.

A typical morning workout can involve dumbbell or kettlebell squats, lunges, shoulder presses, rows, and swings.

Squats and lunges are basic lower-body workouts that may be done with dumbbells or kettlebells.

hamstrings,glutes,calves,They work with the quadriceps

Adding weights to these workouts increases resistance, resulting in increased muscle activation and strength improvements over time.

Shoulder pushes and rows are great upper-body workouts that can be done with dumbbells or kettlebells. They work the shoulders, back, and arms. These exercises enhance posture, shoulder stability, and total upper-body strength.

Kettlebell swings are a dynamic full-body workout that works your hips, glutes, hamstrings, and core. This abrupt exercise not only increases strength but also improves power and cardiovascular fitness, making it an excellent complement to any morning training regimen.

To get the most out of your dumbbell and kettlebell workouts, focus on perfect form and technique. Starting with lesser weights and progressively increasing resistance as strength increases can assist to avoid injury and maintain consistent growth over time.

In addition to strength and muscle-building advantages, early dumbbell and kettlebell workouts can raise metabolism, increase energy levels, and improve mental clarity and attention throughout the day. By including these easy yet powerful workouts in their morning routines, men may set a good tone for the day ahead, supporting long-term health and well-being.

Dumbbell and kettlebell workouts provide guys with a simple and effective approach to begin their mornings with a full-body workout. Individuals may increase their strength, endurance, and general health by adopting a range of workouts that target different muscle groups, putting them in a position for success both in and outside the gym.

Compound Lifts

Compound lifts are the foundation of every good strength training regimen, providing various advantages for muscle growth, strength development, and total functional fitness.

These exercises train many joints and muscle groups simultaneously, making them efficient and effective for increasing strength and muscular gain.

One of the primary benefits of compound lifts is their ability to activate numerous muscle groups at once, allowing for more effective use of time during training.

Squats, deadlifts, bench presses, and overhead presses work vast muscular groups like the legs, back, chest, and shoulders, resulting in increased total muscle activation and growth.

In addition to increasing muscular mass, compound lifts enhance functional strength by simulating real-life motions and improving coordination and stability.

Squats and deadlifts, for example, need perfect form and technique to lift high weights safely, resulting in increased general strength and balance in daily tasks.

Compound lifts have been proven to stimulate the release of hormones like testosterone and growth hormone, which are essential for muscle development and recovery.

This hormonal reaction not only increases muscle growth but also accelerates metabolism and encourages fat loss, making compound lifts perfect for people trying to modify their body composition.

Incorporating compound lifts into a basic morning exercise regimen for men may be quite useful, giving a time-saving technique to improve strength and jumpstart metabolism for the day.

A typical morning workout can involve a combination of compound lifts and mild cardio or mobility exercises to warm up and prepare the body for the day ahead.

For example, a basic morning routine may include:

Squats: three sets of 8-12 repetitions.

Deadlifts: three sets of 6-10 repetitions.

Bench Press: three sets of 8-12 repetitions.

Pull-ups or rows: three sets of six to ten repetitions
Overhead Press: three sets of eight to twelve repetitions

Performing these compound lifts with good form and technique, progressively increasing the weight as strength increases, can result in considerable advantages for muscle growth, strength development, and general fitness.

Additionally, beginning the day with a morning workout may boost energy, enhance mood, and establish a positive tone for the remainder of the day.

Chapter 4: Cardiovascular Workouts

Cardiovascular exercises are essential for overall fitness and heart health,Cardiovascular exercises are essential

Simple morning workouts can help you start the day with energy and vitality. Here is a comprehensive guide on cardiovascular workouts for guys.

Running or Jogging: Put on your sneakers and hit the streets for a short run or jog. Running engages several muscle groups, boosts the heart rate, and increases cardiovascular endurance.

Begin with a moderate distance, gradually increasing the effort and duration as your fitness improves.

Jump Rope: Jumping rope is an inexpensive and effective cardio activity that raises heart rate while improving coordination and agility. Just a few minutes of jumping rope may provide a significant cardiovascular exercise. To keep things interesting, add modifications like double unders or high knees.

cycling: Whether on a stationary bike or on the road, cycling provides a low-impact yet incredibly effective cardiovascular workout. It strengthens the legs, improves endurance, and burns calories. Adjust the resistance or terrain to your fitness level.

Swimming: Get into the pool for a full-body workout that is gentle on your joints. Swimming strengthens the muscles in the arms, legs, and core while providing a cardiovascular workout.

Alternate between freestyle, breaststroke, and backstroke to target different muscle groups.

Stair Climbing: For a tough cardiovascular workout, use your stairs or a neighboring staircase. Climbing stairs works the lower body muscles and increases the heart rate quickly. Begin with a few flights, gradually increasing the number as your stamina develops.

Dance Workouts: Turn on your favorite music and dance your way to cardiovascular health. Dancing boosts heart rate while increasing coordination, balance, and mood. Follow along with online dance classes or simply freestyle to the beat.

Incorporating these simple morning cardiovascular routines into your routine can help improve your heart health, stamina, and overall fitness level. Remember to start cautiously, listen to your body, and be patient for long-term results.

HIIT Sessions

High-intensity interval Training (HIIT) sessions are an efficient and effective approach to adding vigorous exercise into your daily routine. These routines, created exclusively for guys, are intended to increase calorie burn, enhance cardiovascular health, and build strength in a short period.

A typical HIIT workout consists of alternating short bursts of high-intensity exercise with brief intervals of rest or low-intensity activity. This style maintains a raised heart rate throughout the workout, helping you to burn more calories in less time than standard steady-state cardio activities.

Consider including the following HIIT activities into your morning routine to get your day off to a strong start:

Jumping Jacks: Start with a few sets of jumping jacks to warm up your muscles and raise your heart rate.

Burpees: To target numerous muscle groups and burn calories, do a series of burpees that include a squat, plank, push-up, and leap.

High Knees: Run in place while raising your knees as high as possible with each step. This workout improves cardiovascular endurance and develops the leg muscles.

Mountain Climbers: Start in a plank posture and alternate between raising your knees to your chest in a running motion. This exercise focuses on your core, shoulders, and legs.

Squat Jumps: Begin with a squat and surge upwards into a leap before landing softly back into the squat posture. This exercise increases lower-body strength and power.

Plank Jacks: From a plank position, leap your legs wide apart and then back together, keeping your back straight. This workout works your core and increases stability.

Sprint Intervals: If you have access to an outdoor location or a treadmill, include sprint intervals in your workout. Sprint at your utmost effort for 20-30 seconds, then recover with 60 seconds of walking or jogging.

If you're new to HIIT, start softly and increase the intensity as your fitness improves. To get the most out of your HIIT workouts, aim for 20-30 minutes, including a warm-up and cool-down.

With dedication and consistency, including HIIT in your morning routine may help you attain your fitness objectives quickly.

Low-Impact Options

Low-impact solutions provide sustainable alternatives to numerous elements of life, such as transportation and everyday consumption, while limiting environmental harm.

These solutions stress efficiency, conservation, and lower carbon footprints without sacrificing convenience or quality of life.

Low-impact modes of transportation include walking, cycling, and taking public transit. Walking and cycling not only cut pollution, but they also improve physical health.

Public transportation minimizes the number of individual automobiles on the road, resulting in less traffic congestion and air pollution.

Carpooling and ridesharing services result in less emissions per passenger, reducing environmental impact.

Energy use has a huge impact on environmental sustainability. Switching to renewable energy sources such as solar, wind, or hydroelectric power reduces dependency on fossil fuels and lowers greenhouse gas emissions.

Energy-efficient appliances, LED lights, and smart home technologies help to reduce energy use, saving money and resources.

Waste reduction is another critical component of low-impact living. Choosing reusable things like water bottles, shopping bags, and containers helps to limit the usage of single-use plastics.

Composting organic waste diverts it from landfills, enhancing soil and lowering methane emissions. Choosing items with minimum packaging and buying in bulk also helps to decrease waste.

Adopting a plant-based diet or eating less meat can have a major influence on the environment. Plant-based diets use fewer resources, emit fewer pollutants, and contribute to biodiversity conservation.

Supporting local, organic, and seasonal produce minimizes the carbon footprint of food transportation and promotes sustainable agricultural techniques.

Water conservation is critical to sustaining freshwater supplies. Installing water-saving devices such as low-flow toilets and showerheads minimizes water use while maintaining comfort. Collecting rainwater for gardening and landscaping decreases dependency on municipal water supply.

Using eco-friendly materials in building and housing, such as bamboo, repurposed wood, and low-VOC paints, decreases environmental effects. Designing energy-efficient buildings with suitable insulation and passive heating and cooling strategies reduces energy usage.

Choosing low-impact solutions is good not just for the environment, but also for your health and well-being. Individuals may help to ensure a more sustainable future for future generations by making deliberate decisions about transportation, energy use, waste reduction, food consumption, water usage, and building.

Cardio + Bodyweight Circuits

Starting your day with a simple morning workout can help you have more energy, be more productive, and feel better overall.

Incorporating aerobic and bodyweight circuits into your regimen may create a complete exercise that stimulates several muscle groups while getting your heart rate up. Here's a simple approach to aerobic and bodyweight circuits for men:

1. Warm-Up: Start with a five-minute energetic warm-up to prepare your body for exercise. Include arm circles, leg swings, hip rotations, and torso twists to improve blood flow and flexibility.

2. Cardiovascular Exercise: Start with 10-15 minutes of cardio to increase your heart rate and metabolism. Cycling, jumping jacks, jogging in place, and high knees are all options. Choose an activity that you love and can commit to for the duration of the session.

3. ***Bodyweight Circuit:*** Complete bodyweight exercises in a circuit manner, with minimum rest in between. Each of the exercises should be repeated 10-15 times or as much as you can easily perform it.

Push-Ups: Work the chest, shoulders, and triceps. Maintain a straight line from head to heels, and lower your body until your chest is almost touching the ground.

Bodyweight Squats activate the quadriceps, hamstrings, and glutes. Stand with your feet shoulder-width apart, stoop down as if you were sitting in a chair, and then stand back up.

Lunges: Work the lower body muscles such as quadriceps, glutes, and calves. Step forward with one leg, lowering your body until both knees are bent at 90 degrees, then return to the starting position and repeat on the opposite side.

Plank strengthens the core muscles. Maintain a push-up stance with straight arms, engage your core, and keep your body in a straight line from head to heels.

Mountain Climbers: Works the core, shoulders, and legs. Begin in a push-up position and alternately bring each knee to the chest in a running motion.

4. Cool down: After the workout, stretch for five minutes to increase flexibility and minimize muscular pain. Stretch the key muscle groups engaged throughout the workout, holding each stretch for 15–30 seconds.

Incorporate this basic morning workout regimen into your daily schedule to boost your energy and vigor. Adjust the intensity and length of each workout to meet your fitness level and objectives. Maintain consistency and get the rewards of a healthier, more active lifestyle.

Chapter 5: Core Strengthening

Core strengthening is critical for general health and stability, especially for guys looking for a quick morning workout regimen.

A strong core not only improves posture, but it also helps with everyday motions, lowers the chance of injury, and improves sports performance. Here's a thorough guide on core strengthening exercises designed for men's early workouts.

Plank: Begin in a push-up posture, resting your forearms. Maintain a straight line from head to heels while working your core muscles. Hold for 30-60 seconds, progressively increasing the duration as you go.

Russian Twists: Sit on the floor, knees bent and feet flat. Lean back slightly, but maintain your back straight. Hold a weight or medicine ball in both hands and rotate your body from side to side, bringing the weight to the floor alongside you. Aim for 10 to 15 reps per side.

Leg Raises: Lie on your back, arms at your sides. Lift your legs to the ceiling while maintaining them straight until your hips are fully flexed. Slowly drop your legs back down, avoiding letting them touch the floor. Complete 10-15 repetitions with controlled motions.

Dead Bug: Lie on your back, arms stretched to the ceiling, legs bent at a 90-degree angle. Lower one arm and the opposing leg to the floor while keeping touch with the ground. Return to the beginning position, then repeat with the opposing limbs. Aim for 10 to 12 repetitions each side.

Bicycle Crunches: Lie on your back, hands behind your head, legs raised, and knees bent at a 90-degree angle. Bring your right elbow towards your left knee while straightening your right leg, then switch to the other side. Perform 12-15 repetitions per side.

Bird Dog: Beggin on your hands and knees, with wrists under shoulders and knees beneath hips. Extend your right arm forward and your left leg back while keeping your back flat and hips level.

Hold for a few seconds before returning to the start position and switching sides. per side Perform 10 to 12 repetitions

Incorporate these core strengthening exercises into your morning routine to establish a firm foundation of strength and stability. Consistency is essential, so strive to do these exercises 3-4 times a week for best results. Remember to use appropriate form and controlled motions to increase efficacy and limit the chance of harm.

Core Importance

Beginning your day with a basic morning fitness regimen might pave the way for better physical and mental health. Among the many workouts, concentrating on core strength is quite important for guys. Here's why.

Enhanced Stability and Balance: A strong core promotes stability and balance, both of which are necessary for daily activities and injury prevention. Simple workouts such as planks, Russian twists, and bicycle crunches work core muscles and improve general stability.

Improved Posture: Poor posture is a widespread problem, particularly with extended sitting and sedentary lifestyles. Core exercises serve to strengthen the muscles that maintain good posture, lowering the risk of back discomfort and fostering a confident stance.

Functional Strength: Core muscles are essential in practically every activity, from bending and lifting to twisting and reaching. Incorporating core workouts into your morning routine builds functional strength, which translates into improved performance in both daily jobs and sports efforts.

Reduced Risk of Injury: Weak core muscles can cause compensations in other sections of the body, raising the risk of injury, particularly during vigorous activities or sports. Regular core workouts assist rectify imbalances and reduce the likelihood of strains and sprains.

Athletic Performance: Whether you like sports or just want to keep active, a strong core is essential for peak athletic performance. It boosts agility, power, and endurance, helping you to succeed at different activities and achieve your fitness objectives more effectively.

Increased Metabolism: Engaging the core muscles in dynamic activities such as mountain climbers or leg lifts can boost the heart rate and contribute to a higher calorie burn throughout the day. This metabolic surge promotes weight control and general fitness.

Enhanced Breathing and Circulation: A strong core promotes good diaphragmatic breathing, which is essential for optimal oxygen exchange and circulation. This not only increases endurance during exercises, but it also improves general respiratory and cardiovascular function.

Simple core exercises may be easily included into your daily routine with little time or equipment. Just a few minutes of abdominal, obliques, and lower back exercises can provide considerable advantages to men of all fitness levels. Whether before breakfast or as a warm-up for the day, focusing on core strength lays the groundwork for a healthier and more active lifestyle. Begin your day with a focus on your core, and receive the benefits of increased strength, stability, and energy.

Effective Exercises

Effective morning workouts for guys do not have to be difficult to be helpful. Incorporating simple but effective activities into your morning routine can help you gain energy, enhance your mood, and jumpstart your metabolism for the day ahead. Here are some simple workouts to get your day off to a good start:

Jumping Jacks: Begin with a traditional warm-up activity like jumping jacks to increase your heart rate and relax your muscles. Aim for 2-3 sets with 20-30 repetitions.

Bodyweight Squats: Squats are an excellent complex exercise that works numerous muscular groups, including the quadriceps, hamstrings, and glutes. To strengthen your lower body, perform three sets of 10-15 repetitions.

Push-ups are a terrific way to increase upper-body strength and engage your chest, shoulders, and triceps. Aim for 2-3 sets of 10-15 repetitions, varying the effort by altering your hand placement or raising your feet as necessary.

Plank: A plank workout helps to strengthen your core and enhance stability. Hold the stance for 30-60 seconds, keeping a straight line from your head to your heels.

Mountain Climbers: Exercise your core and get your heart rate up with mountain climbers. Aim for 2-3 sets of 20-30 seconds each, changing legs in a dynamic and controlled manner.

Burpees are a total-body workout that combines strength training and aerobics. Perform 2-3 sets of 8-12 repetitions to work your muscles and raise your heart rate.

Lunges are excellent for developing lower-body strength and balance. Alternate legs, aiming for 2-3 sets of 10-12 repetitions for each leg.

Russian Twists: Wrap up your morning workout with a core-strengthening exercise like Russian Twists. Sit on the floor, lean back slightly, and twist your body from side to side while holding a weight or a household item. Aim for two to three sets of 12-15 repetitions on each side.

Remember to listen to your body and adjust the workouts as needed to match your fitness level.

Consistency is essential, so add these workouts into your morning routine at least 3-4 times per week for the greatest results. With devotion and effort, you'll see a difference in your strength, endurance, and general well-being.

Stability Training

Stability training is an essential component of any exercise regimen, especially for men who want to increase their general strength and physical resilience. This type of training focuses on strengthening balance, core strength, and proprioception, all of which are necessary for injury prevention, sports performance, and general health.

Incorporating stability training into a simple morning workout regimen for men can produce big results. A succinct yet effective stability-focused routine may include a variety of exercises targeting different muscle groups and components of balance.

Planks: Start with a simple plank and hold it for 30-60 seconds to stimulate your core muscles. Advance to side planks to target the obliques and enhance stability.

Single-leg balance: For 30 seconds, stand on one leg while maintaining stability and appropriate posture. Switch legs and repeat. This exercise improves proprioception and develops the muscles associated with balance.

Bridges: Lie on your back, legs bent, feet flat on the floor. Lift your hips to the ceiling, using your glutes and core muscles. Hold for 15-30 seconds before lowering back down. This exercise promotes hip and lower back stability while also strengthening the posterior chain.

Bosu ball workouts include dynamic motions like squats, lunges, and overhead presses while standing on a bosu ball. The unstable surface tests stability and engages tiny stabilizing muscles, which aids with general balance and coordination.

Resistance band exercises: Use resistance bands for workouts such as lateral walks, monster walks, and resisted rotations to improve hip stability and develop the muscles surrounding the pelvis and knees.

Balance board exercises: Stand on a balance board and do motions like squats, lunges, and twists to challenge your stability and proprioception.

Consistency is essential in stability training. Aim to do these exercises 2-3 times a week, increasing the intensity and length as your stability improves. Remember to focus on appropriate form and alignment to increase efficacy and limit the chance of injury.

To summarize, including stability training into a basic morning workout regimen for men is a proactive strategy for improving overall fitness and lowering the risk of injury. Individuals may increase their physical resilience and athletic performance by focusing on balance, core strength, and proprioception.

Chapter 6: Cool Down and Recovery

Cool down and recovery are essential parts of any exercise regimen, especially after doing Simple Morning Workouts for Men. While the primary focus of exercise is frequently on the vigorous activity itself, the cool down and recovery phases are also critical for improving performance, reducing injury, and increasing general well-being.

Cooling down after an exercise entails gradually lowering the level of physical exertion. This may involve easy stretches or low-intensity exercises that target the muscles engaged throughout the activity.

Cooling down causes the heart rate to gradually return to resting levels, prevents blood pooling in the extremities, and decreases the probability of post-exercise muscular pain.

Recovery, on the other hand, refers to a larger spectrum of actions that help the body repair and regenerate itself.

This involves being adequately hydrated, recharging with nutritional foods, getting enough rest, and indulging in activities like foam rolling or mild massage to relieve muscle tension.

For men who participate in Simple Morning Workouts, implementing an efficient cool down and recovery plan can dramatically improve the advantages of their workout schedule.

A simple but effective cool down might include five to ten minutes of mild jogging or brisk walking, followed by static stretches for key muscle groups such the quadriceps, hamstrings, calves, and upper body muscles.

After the workout, males should emphasize hydration by restoring fluids lost via perspiration. Drinking water or an electrolyte-containing sports drink can assist restore hydration and improve muscular performance.

Nutrition also plays an important part in the rehabilitation process. Within the first hour following exercise, consuming a balanced breakfast or snack including carbs and protein can assist in replacing glycogen levels while also promoting muscle repair and development.

Proper rest is required for the body to adequately recover from exercise-induced stress. Aim for seven to nine hours of excellent sleep every night to promote optimal recovery and wellness.

Incorporating techniques like foam rolling or mild stretching can help with muscle rehabilitation by increasing blood flow and decreasing muscular tension and pain.

Cool down and recovery are important parts of every exercise regimen, including Simple Morning Workouts for Men. By applying these habits, men may improve their performance, lower their risk of injury, and achieve their overall fitness objectives.

Post-Workout Cool Down

After finishing your morning workout regimen, it's critical to take some time to cool down properly.

This not only assists with muscle healing but also prevents injury and enhances flexibility. Here's a thorough guide to post-workout cool down particularly geared for men's basic morning workouts:

Slow Down: As you approach the finish of your workout, progressively lessen the intensity of your movements. This allows your heart rate to gradually decline, reducing dizziness and pain.

Stretch the primary muscle groups you targeted during your workout. This comprises the hamstrings, quadriceps, calves, chest, back, and shoulders. Hold each stretch for 15-30 seconds, aiming for a soft stretch that does not need too much effort.

Foam rolling can help relieve stress and enhance blood flow to your muscles. Roll back and forth slowly for 1-2 minutes each muscle group.

Hydration: Drinking water or a sports drink will replenish the fluids you lost throughout your workout. Proper hydration is critical to muscle repair and general function.

Breathing Exercises: Deep breathing exercises can assist your body shift from effort to relaxation. Inhale deeply through your nose, filling your lungs with oxygen, then gently exhale through your mouth, concentrating on releasing tension.

Light Cardio: Perform 5-10 minutes of light cardiovascular activity, such as walking or cycling at a low intensity. This progressively reduces your heart rate and removes metabolic waste products from your muscles.

Reflect and Relax: Take time to reflect on your workout and recognize your accomplishments. Use this time to mentally prepare for the day ahead, while letting your body to rest and relax.

Proper Nutrition: Refuel your body with a well-balanced post-workout meal or snack rich in carbs and protein to aid in muscle repair and development.

By implementing these easy yet powerful post-exercise cool down techniques into your morning routine, you may improve your workout outcomes and prepare for a productive day ahead. Remember, consistency is essential for sustaining a healthy and active lifestyle.

Static Stretches

Static stretches are a crucial part of every fitness program, especially for men who want to start their mornings with easy yet effective workouts.

Unlike dynamic stretches, which entail movement, static stretches are done by keeping a precise posture for a predetermined length of time, generally 15 to 60 seconds. These stretches promote flexibility, boost blood flow to the muscles, and lower the chance of injury.

Including static stretches in your morning routine might help your body prepare for the day. Before you start stretching, do a few minutes of gentle aerobics to warm up your muscles.

Concentrate on key muscular groups such as the hamstrings, quadriceps, calves, chest, back, and shoulders.

Begin with a hamstring stretch, sitting on the floor with one leg stretched straight in front of you and the other bent. Reach for your toes while maintaining your back straight and hold the stretch for 15-30 seconds on each side.

Next, perform a quadriceps stretch by standing tall and dragging one foot towards your buttocks while keeping your knees together. Hold for 15–30 seconds before swapping sides.

For calf stretches, face a wall and press your hands against it. Step one foot back, keeping it straight, and press your heel into the ground while leaning slightly forward. Hold for 15-30 seconds, then swap legs.

To extend your chest and shoulders, clasp your hands behind your back and slowly move them away from your body, feeling a stretch across your chest. Hold for 15–30 seconds.

For the back, lay on your back with your knees bent and your feet flat on the ground. Bring one knee to your chest and hold it there with both hands, feeling the stretch in your lower back. Hold for 15–30 seconds before switching legs.

Incorporating these static stretches into your morning routine for men may help increase flexibility, relieve muscular tension, and establish a positive tone for the day.

Remember to listen to your body and never put yourself in distress. Consistent stretching will eventually result in enhanced mobility and general physical well-being.

Recovery Tools

When it comes to living a healthy lifestyle, easy morning workouts for guys are an excellent way to get the day started. However, it is equally crucial to prioritize rehabilitation to avoid burnout and damage. Here are some important recuperation strategies to incorporate into your routine:

A foam roller is a multipurpose tool for relieving muscular tension and increasing flexibility. Rolling over tight muscles increases blood flow and reduces soreness, making it an ideal post-workout recovery strategy.

Massage Ball: Like a foam roller, a massage ball targets particular areas of stress with more accuracy. To relieve pain and enhance mobility, apply it to muscular knots, particularly in the shoulders, back, and legs.

Stretching Strap: Including dynamic and static stretching in your post-workout routine can increase flexibility and lower your risk of injury. A stretching strap can help with deeper stretches, allowing you to target muscles that would be difficult to reach on your own.

Compression garments, such as socks or sleeves, can help in muscle rehabilitation by increasing blood flow and decreasing edema. Wearing compression clothing before or after a workout can help reduce tiredness and discomfort, allowing you to recover faster.

Cold treatment: Ice packs or cold treatment devices can help reduce inflammation and numb painful muscles after strenuous exercise. Cold treatment applied to particular areas of discomfort can speed up healing and reduce post-exercise soreness.

Hydration and Nutrition: Proper hydration and nutrition are critical for recovery. After your workout, restore lost fluids and electrolytes and eat a balanced lunch or snack rich in carbs and protein to assist muscle repair and development.

Do not underestimate the value of relaxation and sleep in the recuperation process. Aim for seven to nine hours of excellent sleep every night to allow your body to repair and renew tissues, so you may wake up feeling energized and ready to face your next workout.

Incorporating these recuperation methods into your routine, along with basic morning exercises for men, can help you improve your performance, lower your chance of injury, and achieve your long-term fitness objectives.

Chapter 7: Nutrition and Hydration

To perform well during morning exercises, men must pay attention to both diet and hydration. Here's a complete guide on properly fuelling your body for optimal results:

1. Pre-workout Nutrition:

Consume a balanced lunch 1-2 hours before your workout that includes carbs, protein, and healthy fats.

Carbohydrates offer energy to your muscles, but protein promotes muscle repair and development.

Choose readily digested items like oatmeal, yogurt, fruit, or whole grain toast with nut butter.

2) *Hydration:*

Start your day by sipping a glass of water to rehydrate after a night's sleep.

Drink an additional 8-16 ounces of water 30 minutes before your activity to guarantee appropriate hydration while exercising.

Avoid drinking too much coffee or sugary drinks, as these can cause dehydration and energy dumps.

3. *During the workout:*

Drink water during your workout to stay hydrated.

Consider using a sports drink to restore electrolytes lost via perspiration during longer or more severe activities.

4. Post-workout nutrition:

Consume a protein and carbohydrate mixture within 30 minutes after finishing your workout to help with muscle repair and glycogen replacement.

Examples include a protein shake with banana, Greek yogurt with berries, and a turkey sandwich on whole grain bread.

5. Meal Timing:

To help with recuperation and muscle building, eat a balanced breakfast with protein, carbs, and healthy fats within 2 hours after finishing your workout.

6. Supplemental Considerations:

Some men may benefit from supplements like creatine, branched-chain amino acids (BCAAs), or electrolyte pills to improve their performance and recuperation.

However, always contact a healthcare expert before incorporating supplements into your regimen.

7. Listen to Your Body:

Everyone's dietary requirements and tolerance levels fluctuate, so consider how different diets and hydration techniques affect your energy and performance.

Adjust your diet and hydration strategy to meet your specific requirements and goals.

Men who prioritize good diet and hydration can improve their morning exercises for improved performance, faster recovery, and overall health and well-being.

Pre-Workout Nutrition

Pre-workout nutrition is critical for boosting performance and outcomes, particularly for easy morning exercises geared at males. This thorough book focuses on delivering clear insights into boosting nutrition for early workouts.

Timing is key. Aim to have a nutritious pre-exercise meal or snack 1-2 hours before your morning workout. This enables proper digestion and energy release when exercising.

Carbs for Energy: Focus on complex carbs such as whole grains, fruits, and vegetables. These give prolonged energy, allowing you to push through your workout without becoming exhausted.

Protein for Muscle Support: Use lean protein sources like eggs, Greek yogurt, or protein drinks. Protein helps with muscle repair and growth, which is crucial for men who want to gain or maintain muscular mass.

Hydration is important: Drink plenty of water before working out. Dehydration can cause poor performance and weariness. Aim to drink at least 16-20 ounces of water 1-2 hours before exercise.

Caffeine Boost: If you tolerate caffeine well, consider taking it before your workout. It improves attention, alertness, and performance. Choose coffee or green tea for a natural energy boost.

Avoid Heavy Fats: While healthy fats are beneficial to general health, eating heavy or fatty foods before working exercise might cause pain and sluggishness. Save these for a post-workout lunch.

Supplements: Depending on your specific needs and goals, try integrating creatine or beta-alanine. However, always contact with a healthcare expert before incorporating supplements into your regimen.

Listen to Your Body: Each person is unique, so pay attention to how your body reacts to different foods and timing methods. Adjust your pre-workout diet to what works best for you.

Post-Workout Nutrition: Do not forget to replenish after your workout. To aid in recuperation and muscle synthesis, have a balanced supper or snack including carbs and protein within 30-60 minutes of your workout.

Consistency is essential for achieving outcomes. To improve performance and reach your fitness objectives, stick to your pre-workout nutrition plan consistently.

Following these simple yet effective pre-workout eating instructions will guarantee that men have the energy and nutrients they need to push through morning exercises and reach their fitness goals.

Post-Workout Fuel

Post-exercise food is essential for refilling energy reserves, promoting muscle repair, and optimizing the advantages of your workout.

For guys who engage in basic morning workouts, choosing the correct nutrition is critical to getting the day started and supporting fitness objectives effectively.

Protein: Following a morning workout, protein is essential for muscle repair and development. Choose sources such as eggs, Greek yogurt, protein drinks, or lean meats like chicken or turkey. Aim for at least 20-30 grams of protein to help with recuperation.

Carbohydrates: Replacing glycogen reserves destroyed during activity is critical for maintaining energy levels. Add complex carbs like whole grains, fruits, and veggies to your post-workout meal. These offer a consistent stream of energy and assist in recuperation.

Hydration: Hydration is often underestimated, although it is essential for peak performance and recuperation. Drinking water or electrolyte-rich drinks after an exercise helps to restore fluids lost via perspiration. Coconut water and sports drinks can assist restore electrolyte balance.

Healthy Fats: Including healthy fats in your post-workout meal will help with nutrient absorption and give lasting energy. For a well-balanced nutritional composition, include nuts, seeds, avocados, or olive oil in your meals.

Timing: To enhance nutritional absorption and muscle repair, replenish within 30 minutes to an hour after your workout. This is the optimal time for your body to restore glycogen reserves and initiate muscle repair.

Avoid Excessive sweets: While carbs are necessary, avoid excessive sweets and processed meals after a workout since they can elevate blood sugar levels and slow recovery. Choose full, nutrient-dense meals instead.

Portion Control: Pay attention to portion sizes to ensure you're getting adequate nutrients without going overboard. Balancing protein, carbs, and fats in the right quantities will help you achieve your fitness objectives without consuming extra calories.

Listen to Your Body: Each person's dietary requirements differ depending on factors such as workout intensity, body composition, and metabolism. Listen to your body's hunger and satiety signals and adapt your post-workout meal accordingly.

Incorporating these principles into your post-workout routine may help you recover faster, build more muscle, and achieve your overall fitness objectives, ensuring that your easy morning exercises for men are both successful and satisfying.

Hydration Guidelines

Proper hydration is essential for peak performance and general health, particularly during easy morning exercises for men. Here are some detailed suggestions to keep you hydrated and invigorated during your workout:

Start hydrated before your workout. Aim to consume 16-20 ounces of water one to two hours before exercise. This ensures your body is well hydrated before you begin sweating.

During Workout Hydration: Drink water often to replenish fluids lost via sweating. The American Council on Exercise suggests drinking 7-10 ounces of water every 10-20 minutes when exercising, depending on intensity, duration, and perspiration rate.

Electrolyte Balance: For longer exercises or in hot weather, try using electrolyte-rich drinks or supplements to restore salt, potassium, and other vital minerals lost via sweating. This promotes adequate fluid balance and prevents dehydration and electrolyte abnormalities.

Post-Workout Rehydration: Drink more water after your workout to restore fluid losses and assist in recovery. Aim to drink at least 16-24 ounces of water for each pound lost while exercising. Including a source of electrolytes in your post-workout water can also help.

Monitor Hydration Status: Look for indicators of dehydration, such as thirst, dark urine, lethargy, dizziness, or headaches. These might signal that you should drink more fluids.

Monitoring your body weight before and after exercise can also help you determine your hydration level—try to limit weight loss during exercises.

Individual Needs: Keep in mind that hydration requirements vary according to body size, perspiration rate, environment, and activity intensity. Listen to your body and modify your hydration intake as needed.

Avoid Overhydration: While being hydrated is important, overhydration can lead to hyponatremia. As a general rule, drink according to your thirst and keep an eye on the color of your urine.

Following these hydration rules can help you improve your performance, recuperation, and general well-being during your basic morning exercises. Remember that consistency is crucial, so prioritize hydration every day.

CONCLUSION

Morning workouts have various benefits for women, including physical, mental, and emotional health. Women may achieve balance and harmony in their lives by taking a holistic approach to health that includes breathwork, mindfulness, and exercise.

First and foremost, morning yoga is an effective technique for improving physical wellness. The exercise promotes flexibility, strength, and balance, which are especially useful to women of all ages.

It helps to relieve tension and promotes good posture, which is crucial for overcoming the sedentary consequences of contemporary lifestyles. Workout's emphasis on mindful movement can also help with menstruation pain and reproductive health, providing women with a natural and holistic approach to well-being.

Morning Workouts promote mental and emotional well-being. Women who practice mindfulness techniques like meditation and deep breathing can reduce stress and improve mental clarity.

This practice promotes self-awareness and compassion, allowing women to face life's adversities with fortitude and grace. Workouts promotes the release of endorphins, which are necessary for emotional balance.

Morning Workouts offer women a holy area for self-care and reflection. Women who set aside time for themselves at the start of each day might set a positive tone for the hours that follow.

This devoted time allows for introspection, goal-setting, and intention-setting, generating a sense of power and purpose. The communal component of yoga provides women with a supporting network of like-minded people, encouraging connection and camaraderie.

Morning Workouts is a transforming practice that enables women to nourish their mind, body, and soul. By adopting this ancient practice, women may build a feeling of balance, resilience, and joy in their lives.

 Morning workout, whether performed alone or in a group setting, provides a sanctuary of calm and empowerment, bringing women to a life of health and purpose.

THANK YOU PAGE

Thank you for selecting this book. Your support is really appreciated. Similarly, I am grateful for the purchase of this book.

Your input is valuable; please share your ideas in a review. It serves as a reference for future improvements. Enjoy reading and utilizing it!

*Workout planner
to help track
progress and
improvements
over time*

Weekly

Sunday

Monday

Tuesday

Goals

Goals

Goals

Wednesday

Thursday

Friday

Goals

Goals

Goals

Saturday

Goals

Mood

Motivation ________________________________
____
____
____
____

Weekly

Week : ______________

Month: ______________

Sunday

Monday

Tuesday

Goals

Goals

Goals

Wednesday

Thursday

Friday

Goals

Goals

Goals

Saturday

Goals

Mood

Motivation ____________________

____

____

____

____

Weekly

Workout Planner

Week :____________

Month: ____________

Sunday

Monday

Tuesday

Goals

Goals

Goals

Wednesday

Thursday

Friday

Goals

Goals

Goals

Saturday

Goals

Mood

Motivation ____________

Weekly

Sunday

Monday

Tuesday

Goals

Goals

Goals

Wednesday

Thursday

Friday

Goals

Goals

Goals

Saturday

Goals

Mood

Motivation

Weekly

Workout Planner

Week : _____________

Month: _____________

Sunday

Monday

Tuesday

Goals

Goals

Goals

Wednesday

Thursday

Friday

Goals

Goals

Goals

Saturday

Goals

Mood

Motivation _______________________________

____

____

____

____

Weekly

Week : _______________

Month: _______________

Sunday

Monday

Tuesday

Goals

Goals

Goals

Wednesday

Thursday

Friday

Goals

Goals

Goals

Saturday

Goals

Mood

Motivation

Weekly

Workout Planner

Week :___________________

Month: ___________________

Sunday

Monday

Tuesday

| Goals | Goals | Goals |

Wednesday

Thursday

Friday

| Goals | Goals | Goals |

Saturday

| Goals | Mood |

Motivation __________________________

Weekly

Week: ___________

Month: ___________

Sunday

Monday

Tuesday

Goals

Goals

Goals

Wednesday

Thursday

Friday

Goals

Goals

Goals

Saturday

Goals

Mood

Motivation

Weekly

Workout Planner

Week : _______________

Month: _______________

Sunday

Monday

Tuesday

Goals

Goals

Goals

Wednesday

Thursday

Friday

Goals

Goals

Goals

Saturday

Goals

Mood

Motivation _______________

![Running figure icon] **Weekly** Workout Planner

Week :_______________

Month:_______________

Sunday

Monday

Tuesday

Goals

Goals

Goals

Wednesday

Thursday

Friday

Goals

Goals

Goals

Saturday

Goals

Mood

Motivation _______________

Weekly

Week :_______________

Month: _______________

Sunday

Monday

Tuesday

Goals

Goals

Goals

Wednesday

Thursday

Friday

Goals

Goals

Goals

Saturday

Goals

Mood

Motivation _______________

Weekly

Sunday

Monday

Tuesday

Goals

Goals

Goals

Wednesday

Thursday

Friday

Goals

Goals

Goals

Saturday

Goals

Mood

Motivation

Weekly
Workout Planner
Week :
Month:
Sunday
Monday
Tuesday
Goals
Goals
Goals
Wednesday
Thursday
Friday
Goals
Goals
Goals
Saturday
Goals
Mood
Motivation

Weekly
Workout Planner
Week :
Month:
Sunday
Monday
Tuesday
Goals
Goals
Goals
Wednesday
Thursday
Friday
Goals
Goals
Goals
Saturday
Goals
Mood
Motivation

Weekly

Workout Planner

Week :_______________

Month: _______________

Sunday

Monday

Tuesday

Goals

Goals

Goals

Wednesday

Thursday

Friday

Goals

Goals

Goals

Saturday

Goals

Mood

Motivation _______________________

Weekly

Workout Planner

Week : _______________

Month: _______________

Sunday

Monday

Tuesday

Goals

Goals

Goals

Wednesday

Thursday

Friday

Goals

Goals

Goals

Saturday

Goals

Mood

Motivation _______________________________

Weekly

Workout Planner

Week :_______________

Month: _______________

Sunday

Monday

Tuesday

Goals

Goals

Goals

Wednesday

Thursday

Friday

Goals

Goals

Goals

Saturday

Goals

Mood

Motivation

Weekly

Workout Planner

Week:_____________

Month:_____________

Sunday

Monday

Tuesday

Goals

Goals

Goals

Wednesday

Thursday

Friday

Goals

Goals

Goals

Saturday

Goals

Mood

Motivation ___________________________________

Workout Planner

Weekly

Week :______________

Month: ______________

Sunday

Monday

Tuesday

Goals

Goals

Goals

Wednesday

Thursday

Friday

Goals

Goals

Goals

Saturday

Goals

Mood

Motivation ________________________

Weekly
Workout Planner
Week :_______________
Month:_______________
Sunday
Monday
Tuesday
Goals
Goals
Goals
Wednesday
Thursday
Friday
Goals
Goals
Goals
Saturday
Goals
Mood
Motivation

Weekly

Sunday　　　　Monday　　　　Tuesday

Goals　　　　Goals　　　　Goals

Wednesday　　　　Thursday　　　　Friday

Goals　　　　Goals　　　　Goals

Saturday

Goals　　　　Mood

Motivation

Weekly

Workout Planner

Week : _______________

Month: _______________

Sunday

Monday

Tuesday

Goals

Goals

Goals

Wednesday

Thursday

Friday

Goals

Goals

Goals

Saturday

Goals

Mood

Motivation ________________________

Weekly

Workout Planner

Week:_____________

Month:_____________

Sunday

Monday

Tuesday

Goals

Goals

Goals

Wednesday

Thursday

Friday

Goals

Goals

Goals

Saturday

Goals

Mood

Motivation _______________________

____
____
____
____

Weekly

Workout Planner

Week :_______________

Month: _______________

Sunday   Monday   Tuesday

| Goals | Goals | Goals |

Wednesday   Thursday   Friday

| Goals | Goals | Goals |

Saturday

| Goals | Mood |

Motivation ___________________________

____

____

____

____

Weekly

Workout Planner

Week: _______________

Month: _______________

Sunday

Monday

Tuesday

Goals

Goals

Goals

Wednesday

Thursday

Friday

Goals

Goals

Goals

Saturday

Goals

Mood

Motivation _______________

![stick figure running] **Weekly** Workout Planner

Week :_______________

Month: _______________

Sunday   Monday   Tuesday

| Goals | Goals | **Goals** |

Wednesday   Thursday   Friday

| Goals | **Goals** | Goals |

Saturday

| Goals | Mood |

Motivation _______________________________
____
____
____
____

Weekly

Week : _______________

Month: _______________

Sunday

Monday

Tuesday

Goals

Goals

Goals

Wednesday

Thursday

Friday

Goals

Goals

Goals

Saturday

Goals

Mood

Motivation _______________

Weekly

Workout Planner

Week : _______________

Month: _______________

Sunday

Monday

Tuesday

Goals

Goals

Goals

Wednesday

Thursday

Friday

Goals

Goals

Goals

Saturday

Goals

Mood

Motivation _______________

Weekly

Workout Planner

Week : _______________

Month: _______________

Sunday

Monday

Tuesday

Goals

Goals

Goals

Wednesday

Thursday

Friday

Goals

Goals

Goals

Saturday

Goals

Mood

Motivation _______________________________

Weekly

Workout Planner

Week : _____________

Month: _____________

Sunday

Monday

Tuesday

Goals

Goals

Goals

Wednesday

Thursday

Friday

Goals

Goals

Goals

Saturday

Goals

Mood

Motivation _______________________________

Weekly

Week : _____________

Month: _____________

Sunday

Monday

Tuesday

Goals

Goals

Goals

Wednesday

Thursday

Friday

Goals

Goals

Goals

Saturday

Goals

Mood

Motivation _______________________

![runner icon] # Weekly **Workout Planner**

Week : _______________

Month: _______________

Sunday	Monday	Tuesday
Goals	Goals	**Goals**

Wednesday	Thursday	Friday
Goals	**Goals**	Goals

Saturday

Goals	Mood 😖 😊 😌 😁 😞

Motivation _______________________________

____

____

____

____

Weekly

Workout Planner

Week: ___________

Month: ___________

Sunday	Monday	Tuesday
Goals	Goals	Goals

Wednesday	Thursday	Friday
Goals	Goals	Goals

Saturday

Goals

Mood

Motivation __________________

____

____

____

____

Weekly

Sunday

Monday

Tuesday

Goals

Goals

Goals

Wednesday

Thursday

Friday

Goals

Goals

Goals

Saturday

Goals

Mood

Motivation _______________________________

Weekly

Workout Planner

Week : _______________

Month: _______________

Sunday

Monday

Tuesday

Goals

Goals

Goals

Wednesday

Thursday

Friday

Goals

Goals

Goals

Saturday

Goals

Mood

Motivation _______________
____
____
____
____

Weekly

Workout Planner

Week :_____________

Month: _____________

Sunday

Monday

Tuesday

Goals

Goals

Goals

Wednesday

Thursday

Friday

Goals

Goals

Goals

Saturday

Goals

Mood

Motivation

Weekly

Workout Planner

Week :___________

Month:___________

Sunday

Monday

Tuesday

| Goals | Goals | **Goals** |

Wednesday

Thursday

Friday

| Goals | **Goals** | Goals |

Saturday

| Goals | Mood |

Motivation _______________

Weekly

Sunday   Monday   Tuesday

Goals   Goals   **Goals**

Wednesday   Thursday   Friday

Goals   **Goals**   Goals

Saturday

Goals   Mood

Motivation

Weekly

Workout Planner

Week :_______________

Month: _______________

Sunday

Monday

Tuesday

Goals

Goals

Goals

Wednesday

Thursday

Friday

Goals

Goals

Goals

Saturday

Goals

Mood

Motivation ______________________________

![running figure]

Weekly

Workout Planner

Week :_______________

Month: _______________

Sunday   Monday   Tuesday

Goals   Goals   Goals

Wednesday   Thursday   Friday

Goals   Goals   Goals

Saturday

Goals   Mood

Motivation ________________________________
____
____
____
____

Workout Planner

Weekly

Week :______________

Month: ______________

Sunday

Monday

Tuesday

| Goals | Goals | **Goals** |

Wednesday

Thursday

Friday

| Goals | **Goals** | Goals |

Saturday

| Goals | Mood |

Motivation

Weekly

Workout Planner

Week : _______________

Month: _______________

Sunday

Monday

Tuesday

Goals

Goals

Goals

Wednesday

Thursday

Friday

Goals

Goals

Goals

Saturday

Goals

Mood

Motivation _______________

Weekly

Workout Planner

Week :_______________

Month: _______________

Sunday

Monday

Tuesday

Goals

Goals

Goals

Wednesday

Thursday

Friday

Goals

Goals

Goals

Saturday

Goals

Mood

Motivation _______________

Weekly

Week: _____________

Month: _____________

Sunday

Monday

Tuesday

Goals

Goals

Goals

Wednesday

Thursday

Friday

Goals

Goals

Goals

Saturday

Goals

Mood

Motivation _______________

Weekly
Workout Planner
Week :_____________
Month:_____________
Sunday
Monday
Tuesday
Goals
Goals
Goals
Wednesday
Thursday
Friday
Goals
Goals
Goals
Saturday
Goals
Mood
Motivation

Weekly
Workout Planner

Week :_______________

Month: _______________

Sunday   Monday   Tuesday

| Goals | Goals | Goals |

Wednesday   Thursday   Friday

| Goals | Goals | Goals |

Saturday

| Goals | Mood |

Motivation ________________________________

____

____

____

Weekly

Workout Planner

Week: _______________

Month: _______________

Sunday

Monday

Tuesday

Goals

Goals

Goals

Wednesday

Thursday

Friday

Goals

Goals

Goals

Saturday

Goals

Mood

Motivation _______________

Weekly

Workout Planner

Week : _______________

Month: _______________

Sunday

Monday

Tuesday

Goals

Goals

Goals

Wednesday

Thursday

Friday

Goals

Goals

Goals

Saturday

Goals

Mood

Motivation ________________________

Weekly

Workout Planner

Week :______________

Month: ______________

Sunday

Monday

Tuesday

Goals

Goals

Goals

Wednesday

Thursday

Friday

Goals

Goals

Goals

Saturday

Goals

Mood

Motivation ________________________________
____
____
____

Weekly

Workout Planner

Week : _____________

Month: _____________

Sunday

Monday

Tuesday

Goals

Goals

Goals

Wednesday

Thursday

Friday

Goals

Goals

Goals

Saturday

Goals

Mood

Motivation _________________________

![runner icon] **Workout Planner**

Weekly

Week : ________________

Month: ________________

Sunday

Monday

Tuesday

| Goals | Goals | **Goals** |

Wednesday

Thursday

Friday

| Goals | **Goals** | Goals |

Saturday

| Goals | Mood 😣 😊 🙂 😁 😟 |

Motivation ________________________________

____

____

____

Weekly

Week : ___________

Month: ___________

Sunday

Monday

Tuesday

Goals

Goals

Goals

Wednesday

Thursday

Friday

Goals

Goals

Goals

Saturday

Goals

Mood

Motivation ___________________________

Weekly
Workout Planner

Week : _______________

Month: _______________

Sunday

Monday

Tuesday

Goals

Goals

Goals

Wednesday

Thursday

Friday

Goals

Goals

Goals

Saturday

Goals

Mood

Motivation _______________

Weekly

Workout Planner

Week : _______________

Month: _______________

Sunday   Monday   Tuesday

| Goals | Goals | Goals |

Wednesday   Thursday   Friday

| Goals | Goals | Goals |

Saturday

| Goals | Mood |

Motivation ________________________

Weekly

Workout Planner

Week : _______________

Month: _______________

Sunday

Goals

Monday

Goals

Tuesday

Goals

Wednesday

Goals

Thursday

Goals

Friday

Goals

Saturday

Goals

Mood

Motivation ___________________________

____

____

____

Weekly

Workout Planner

Week : _______________

Month: _______________

Sunday

Monday

Tuesday

| Goals | Goals | **Goals** |

Wednesday

Thursday

Friday

| Goals | **Goals** | Goals |

Saturday

| Goals | Mood |

Motivation _______________________________________

____

____

____

Weekly

Workout Planner

Week :_______________

Month: _______________

Sunday	Monday	Tuesday
Goals	Goals	Goals

Wednesday	Thursday	Friday
Goals	Goals	Goals

Saturday	Mood
Goals	

Motivation ___________________________

Weekly

Workout Planner

Week :_____________

Month:_____________

Sunday

Monday

Tuesday

Goals

Goals

Goals

Wednesday

Thursday

Friday

Goals

Goals

Goals

Saturday

Goals

Mood

Motivation _______________

Weekly

Workout Planner

Week : _______________

Month: _______________

Sunday   Monday   Tuesday

Goals   Goals   Goals

Wednesday   Thursday   Friday

Goals   Goals   Goals

Saturday

Goals   Mood

Motivation

Workout Planner
Weekly
Week :
Month:
Sunday
Monday
Tuesday
Goals
Goals
Goals
Wednesday
Thursday
Friday
Goals
Goals
Goals
Saturday
Goals
Mood
Motivation

Weekly

Workout Planner

Week :________________

Month:________________

Sunday

Monday

Tuesday

Goals

Goals

Goals

Wednesday

Thursday

Friday

Goals

Goals

Goals

Saturday

Goals

Mood

Motivation ____________________________

Weekly

Workout Planner

Week : _______________

Month: _______________

Sunday   Monday   Tuesday

| Goals | Goals | Goals |

Wednesday   Thursday   Friday

| Goals | Goals | Goals |

Saturday

| Goals | Mood |

Motivation ___________________________________

____

____

____

Weekly

Workout Planner

Week :________________

Month: ________________

Sunday

Monday

Tuesday

Goals

Goals

Goals

Wednesday

Thursday

Friday

Goals

Goals

Goals

Saturday

Goals

Mood

Motivation

Weekly
Workout Planner
Week :
Month:
Sunday
Monday
Tuesday
Goals
Goals
Goals
Wednesday
Thursday
Friday
Goals
Goals
Goals
Saturday
Goals
Mood
Motivation

Workout Planner
Weekly
Week :
Month:
Sunday
Monday
Tuesday
Goals
Goals
Goals
Wednesday
Thursday
Friday
Goals
Goals
Goals
Saturday
Goals
Mood
Motivation